# Plant Based Instant Pot Cookbook

*Healthy and Low Carb Recipes to Lose Weight and Jumpstart your Health Following a Vegan Diet*

**July Kern**

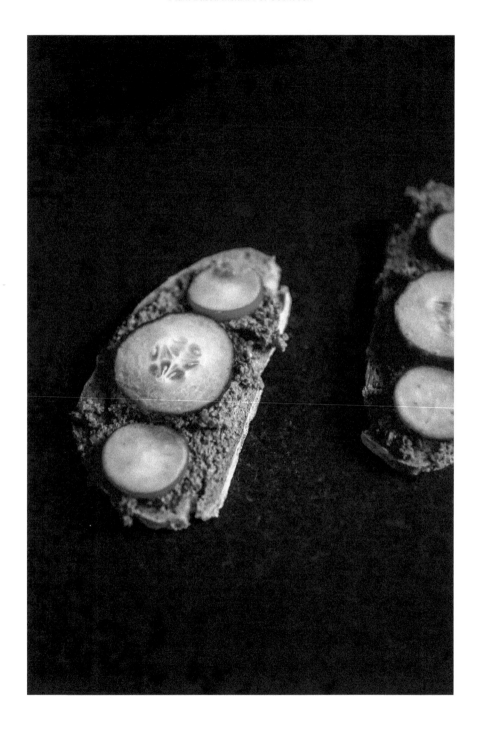

# Table Of Contents

**INTRODUCTION** ........................................................................ **8**

**BREAKFAST** ............................................................................ **10**

    1.   OATMEAL MUFFINS ........................................................ 10

    2.   TEMPEH BOWL ............................................................. 12

    3.   TENDER TOFU CUBES ..................................................... 15

    4.   POTATO PANCAKES ....................................................... 17

    5.   AVOCADO SANDWICHES .................................................. 19

**BURGERS AND PATTIES** ........................................................ **22**

    6.   CRANBERRY PATTIES ..................................................... 22

    7.   SWEET PEAR PATTIES .................................................... 25

    8.   MASHED WHITE POTATO PATTIES ..................................... 27

    9.   LEEK PATTIES ............................................................. 29

    10.   ASPARAGUS BURGER ..................................................... 31

**SIDE DISHES** ......................................................................... **34**

    11.   PASTA AND GREEN PEAS SIDE DISH ................................... 34

    12.   ALMOND MILK MILLET .................................................. 36

    13.   STIR FRIED KALE ......................................................... 37

    14.   ZOODLES ................................................................... 39

    15.   BUCKWHEAT ............................................................... 41

**GRAINS AND PASTA** .............................................................. **44**

    16.   CREAMY SPELT BERRIES ................................................ 44

    17.   BULGUR SALAD ........................................................... 46

    18.   VEGAN QUINOA PILAF ................................................... 48

    19.   RICE GARDEN SALAD .................................................... 50

    20.   LEMON PASTA ............................................................. 52

**BEANS AND LENTILS** ....................................................**56**

21.   LENTIL RAGOUT .............................................. 56

22.   LENTIL MASH.................................................... 59

23.   RED LENTIL DAL .............................................. 61

24.   LENTIL TOMATO SALAD ................................ 63

25.   CABBAGE ROLLS WITH LENTILS .................... 65

**SOUP AND STEWS** .......................................................**68**

26.   SUMMER STEW ............................................... 68

27.   TEXAS STEW ................................................... 70

28.   SOYBEAN STEW............................................... 72

29.   IRANIAN STEW ................................................ 74

30.   RATSHERRENPFANNE ...................................... 76

**MAIN DISHES** .............................................................**78**

31.   STUFFED MINI PUMPKINS ............................... 78

32.   NUT LOAF ........................................................ 81

33.   FRAGRANT SPRING ONIONS ........................... 85

34.   BEET STEAKS .................................................. 87

35.   STUFFED FIGS.................................................. 90

**SNACKS AND APPETIZERS** .......................................**94**

36.   CRUNCHY ARTICHOKE HEARTS ..................... 94

37.   SCALLION PANCAKES ...................................... 96

38.   MUSHROOM ARANCINI .................................... 98

39.   COATED HEART OF PALM ............................. 101

40.   SWEET TOFU CUBES ..................................... 103

**SAUCES AND FILLINGS** ............................................................. **106**

    41.    ROASTED PEPPER SALSA ................................................. 106

    42.    ARUGULA HUMMUS ...................................................... 109

    43.    EDAMOLE ................................................................... 111

    44.    PIZZA SAUCE .............................................................. 113

    45.    GARLIC DIP................................................................. 115

**DESSERTS** .............................................................................. **118**

    46.    CREAM PIE PUDDING.................................................... 118

    47.    BANANA CAKE............................................................ 121

    48.    CARAMBOLA IN CHAI SYRUP......................................... 123

    49.    SEMOLINA PUDDING WITH MANGO................................... 125

    50.    WALNUT SWEETS......................................................... 127

**CONCLUSION**........................................................................... **130**

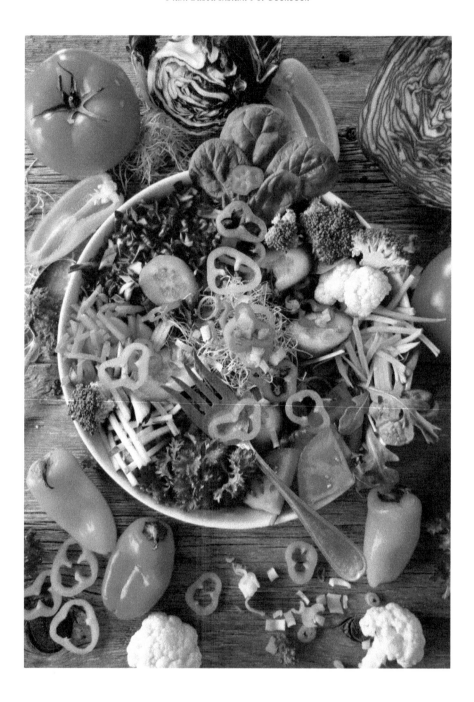

# Introduction

Nowadays veganism is one of the most popular trends all over the world. Thousands of people prefer to refuse animal products and follow a natural lifestyle. A vegan diet has started its history since the 1944 year and in five years later Leslie J Cross suggested to get the definition for veganism. He supported the idea of the emancipation of animals from the human's exploitation. During the years the definition of veganism had been modified and now it became the lifestyle which supports respectful attitude to animals and nature in general.

Veganism is the type of vegetarianism which implies the restriction of meat, poultry, seafood, and dairy products. What do vegans eat? The vegan diet is very diverse. There are a million recipes that can satisfy the most demanded tastes. Cakes, pastries, pies, stews, curries – each of this meal is included in a vegan diet. There is only one condition: every meal should be cooked from plant-based ingredients. Vegans get all the vital vitamins, minerals, and proteins from vegetables, fruits, grains, nuts, and seeds.

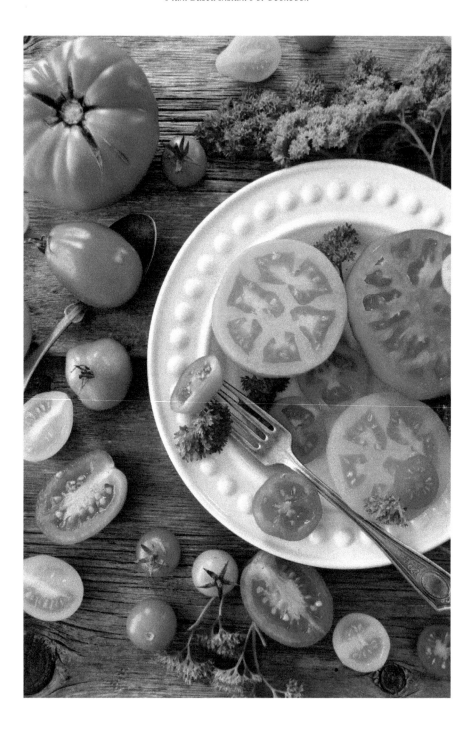

# Breakfast

## 1. Oatmeal Muffins

**Prep:** 10 minutes **Cooking:** 8 minutes**Servings:** 6

**Ingredients:**

- 1 cup quick oats 2 tablespoon white sugar

- 1 teaspoon vanilla extract

- ¼ cup wheat flour 1 teaspoon almond butter

- 2 tablespoon coconut milk

- 1 oz walnuts, chopped

- Cooking spray

**Directions:**

1. In the mixing bowl combine together dry ingredients: whitesugar, quick oats, wheat flour, and chopped walnuts.

2. Mix up the mixture well and add almond butter, vanilla extract,and coconut milk.

3. Stir the mixture with the help of a spoon.

4. Spray muffin molds with the cooking spray.

5. Scoop the oat mixture in the molds and press gently.

6. Cover the molds with foil and pin it with the help of a toothpick.

7. Transfer it in the instant pot bowl and close the lid.

8. Cook muffins on High (Manual mode) for 8 minutes. Use quickpressure release.

**Nutrition value/serving:** calories 145, fat 6.4, fiber 2.2, carbs 18.6, protein4.2

# 2. Tempeh Bowl

**Prep time:** 10 minutes **Cooking time:** 11 minutes

**Servings:** 5

**Ingredients:**

- ½ cup potatoes, chopped

- 1 cup spinach, chopped

- ½ cup of water

- 1 teaspoon Italian seasoning

- 1 teaspoon sriracha

- 1 tablespoon soy sauce

- 1 teaspoon minced garlic

- 1 teaspoon salt

- 8 oz tempeh, chopped

- ½ cup kale, chopped

- 1 teaspoon nutritional yeast

## Directions:

1. In the mixing bowl mix up together salt, Italian seasoning, andchopped potato.

2. Insert the steamer rack in the instant pot bowl.

3. Place the potatoes and water in the bottom of the instant potbowl.

4. Then take round instant pot pan and place tempeh inside.

5. Add sriracha, soy sauce, and minced garlic. Mix it up.

6. Then add kale and spinach.

7. Sprinkle the greens with nutritional yeast and cover with foil. Make the pins in the foil with the help of a knife or toothpick.

8. Place the pan on the steamer rack and close the instant pot lid.

9. Cook the meal for 11 minutes on Manual mode (High pressure).

10.        Then make quick pressure release.

11.        Place the meal in the bowls by layers: the layer of potatoes, then greens, and then tempeh.

**Nutrition value/serving:** calories 111, fat 5.3, fiber 0.8, carbs 8.6, protein 9.6

# 3. Tender Tofu Cubes

**Prep time:** 10 minutes **Cooking time:** 15 minutes

**Servings:** 4

**Ingredients:**

- 15 oz firm tofu, cubed

- 1 teaspoon curry powder

- ½ teaspoon salt

- 1 teaspoon garlic powder

- ½ onion, diced

- 1 teaspoon smoked paprika

- 1 teaspoon almond butter

- 1 cup of coconut yogurt

**Directions:**

1. Preheat instant pot bowl on Saute mode.

2. When it shows "hot" toss almond butter

inside.

3. Melt it and add diced onion, garlic powder, salt, curry powder,and smoked paprika.

4. Stir the ingredients and saute for 2 minutes on Saute mode.

5. Then add firm tofu cubes and mix up well.

6. Close the lid and set Manual mode (High pressure). Cook tofu for 2 minutes and them use natural pressure release for 10 minutes.

7. Open the lid and add coconut yogurt. Mix up the meal very well.

8. Place meal in the bowls and serve when it reaches roomtemperature.

**Nutrition value/serving:** calories 185, fat 10.3, fiber 2.3, carbs 12.2,protein 13.5

# 4. Potato Pancakes

**Prep time:** 8 minutes **Cooking time:** 15 minutes

**Servings:** 4

**Ingredients:**

- 3 potatoes, peeled

- 2 tablespoon wheat flour

- 1 teaspoon cornstarch

- 1 teaspoon salt

- ½ teaspoon ground black pepper

- 1 tablespoon chives

- 1 teaspoon fresh dill, chopped

- 1 tablespoon olive oil

**Directions:**

1. Grate potatoes and mix them up with wheat flour, cornstarch, salt. Ground black

pepper, chives, and fresh dill.

2. Separate the mixture into 4 parts.

3. Preheat instant pot bowl till it shows "hot", and pour olive oilinside.

4. Place the first part of grated potato mixture in the instant pot bowl and flatten it to make the shape of a pancake.

5. Cook it on Saute mode for 4 minutes from each side or until"pancake" is light brown.

6. Repeat the same steps with all remaining grated potato mixture.

**Nutrition value/serving:** calories 159, fat 3.7, fiber 4.1, carbs 29, protein

3.2

# 5. Avocado Sandwiches

**Prep time:** 10 minutes **Cooking time:** 6 minutes

**Servings:** 2

**Ingredients:**

- 4 vegan bread slices

- 1 avocado, peeled

- 1 teaspoon minced garlic

- 1 tomato, chopped

- 1 tablespoon coconut oil

- 1 tablespoon chives, chopped

- 1 teaspoon smoked paprika

**Directions:**

1. Mash the avocado with the help of fork and transfer in theblender.

2. Add minced garlic, chopped tomato,

chives, and smokedpaprika.

3. Blend the mixture until smooth.

4. Then spread each bread slice with avocado mixture and makesandwiches.

5. Preheat the instant pot until it shows "Hot".

6. Place the coconut oil inside instant pot bowl and add avocadosandwiches.

7. Set Saute mode and cook them for 3 minutes from each side. Cooked sandwiches should have a light crunchy texture.

**Nutrition value/serving:** calories 326, fat 27.3, fiber 8.1, carbs 20.6,

protein 4.

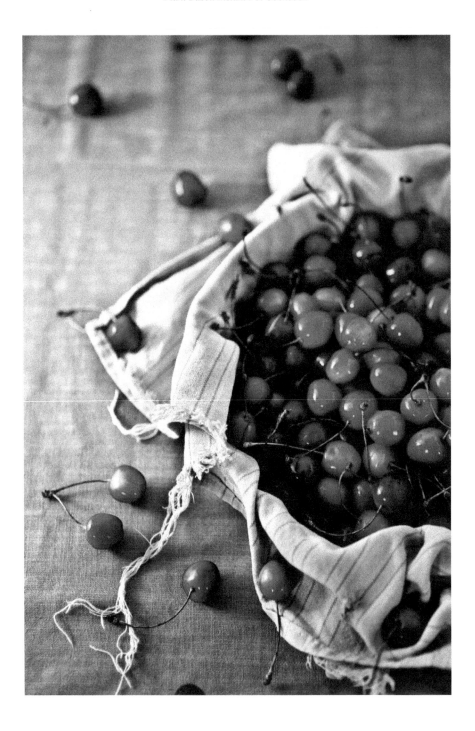

# Burgers and Patties

## 6. Cranberry Patties

**Prep time:** 10 minutes **Cooking time:** 7 minutes

**Servings:** 6

**Ingredients:**

- 1 ½ cup quinoa

- 3 cups of water

- ¼ cup dried cranberries, chopped

- 1/2 cup silken tofu, pureed

- 3 tablespoons wheat flour

- 2 tablespoons fresh dill, chopped

- ¾ teaspoon dried sage

- ½ cup chickpeas, cooked

- Cooking spray

## Directions:

1. Combine together water and quinoa and place in the instant pot.

2. Close the lid and cook on High for 1 minute. Allow natural pressure release for 5 minutes.

3. Transfer the cooked quinoa in the big bowl.

4. Blend chickpeas until smooth and add in the big bowl too.

5. Then add fresh dill, pureed tofu, cranberries, wheat flour, anddried sage.

6. Stir the mass with the spoon and form patties.

7. Spray instant pot with cooking spray and

place patties.

8. Cook them on Saute mode for 3 minutes from each side.

**Nutrition value/serving:** calories 245, fat 4.1, fiber 6.3, carbs 41.7, protein 10.8

# 7. Sweet Pear Patties

**Prep time:** 10 minutes **Cooking time:** 6 minutes

**Servings:** 3

**Ingredients:**

- 1 pear, grated

- ¾ cup almond milk

- ½ cup wheat flour

- 1 tablespoon white sugar

- ½ teaspoon ground cinnamon

- ¾ teaspoon ground cardamom

- 1 teaspoon almond butter

**Directions:**

1. Place all the ingredients except almond butter in the mixingbowl.

2. With the help mix up the mass until

homogenous.

3. Preheat instant pot on Saute mode and add almond butter.

4. Use 2 spoons to make patties from pear mixture. Transfer themin the hot almond butter.

5. Cook sweet patties for 2.5 minutes from one side and then fliponto another side and cook for 2 minutes more.

**Nutrition value/serving:** calories 291, fat 17.6, fiber 4.2, carbs 31.9,

protein 4.9

# 8. Mashed White Potato Patties

**Prep time:** 10 minutes **Cooking time:** 8 minutes

**Servings:** 4

**Ingredients:**

- 3 white potatoes, mashed

- ¼ cup cauliflower, cooked

- ¼ cup flax meal

- 1 teaspoon salt

- 4 tablespoons bread crumbs

- 1 teaspoon dried rosemary

- 1 tablespoon olive oil

**Directions:**

1. Mash cauliflower and mix it up with potatoes, flax meal, salt, and dried rosemary.

2. Make patties and coat them in bread

crumb. Press the patties gently and place in the instant pot.

3. Add olive oil and close the lid.

4. Saute patties for 8 minutes.

5. The cooked patties should have one golden brown side.

**Nutrition value/serving:** calories 199, fat 6.6, fiber 6.4, carbs 32.5, protein 5.2

# 9. Leek Patties

**Prep time:** 10 minutes **Cooking time:** 10 minutes

**Servings:** 2

**Ingredients:**

- 2 cups leek, chopped

- 1 teaspoon olive oil

- 1 tablespoon almond butter

- ¾ cup of water

- 1 tablespoon garam masala

- ¼ cup silken tofu, pureed

- 2 tablespoons rice flour

- 1 teaspoon salt

**Directions:**

1. Put leeks, almond butter, water, and salt in the instant pot.

2. Close the lid and cook the mixture on High for 2 minutes. Then make quick pressure release.

3. Transfer the mass in the bowl and mash gently with the help of a fork.

4. Add garam masala, rice flour, tofu, and mix up well.

5. Make patties and place them in instant pot.

6. Add olive oil and cook them on Saute mode for 4 minutes from each side or until light brown.

**Nutrition value/serving:** calories 172, fat 7.8, fiber 2.7, carbs 22.5, protein 5.1

# 10.    Asparagus Burger

**Prep time:** 10 minutes **Cooking time:** 10 minutes

**Servings:** 4

**Ingredients:**

- 1-pound asparagus

- 1 cup of water

- 1 tablespoon salt

- ½ cup bread crumbs

- 1 teaspoon chili flakes

- 1 teaspoon minced garlic

- ¾ cup fresh parsley, chopped

- 1 teaspoon olive oil

**Directions:**

1. Put asparagus and water in the instant pot.

Add salt and cook iton High for 3 minutes.

2. Then use quick pressure release.

3. Drain water from asparagus and transfer in the blender.

4. Blend until smooth.

5. Mix up together blended asparagus, bread crumbs, chili flakes,minced garlic, and parsley.

6. When you get homogenous mass – make burgers.

7. Preheat instant pot on Saute mode for 5 minutes.

8. Add olive oil and place burgers.

9. Cook burgers for 2 minutes from each side.

**Nutrition value/serving:** calories 91, fat 2.1, fiber 3.4, carbs 15.1, protein4.7

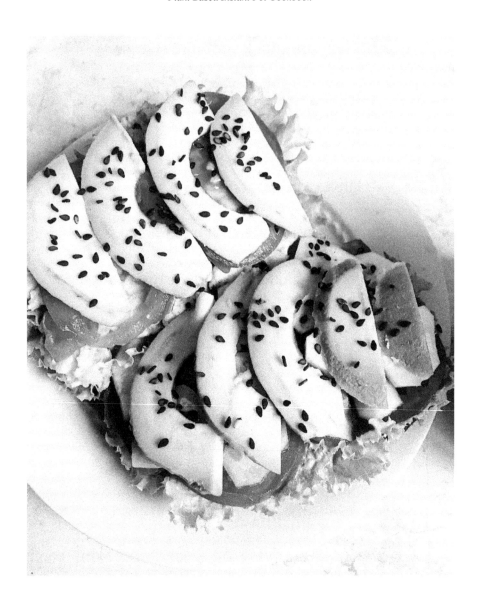

# Side Dishes

## 11.    Pasta and Green Peas Side Dish

**Prep time:** 5 minutes **Cooking time:** 10 minutes

**Servings:** 2

**Ingredients:**

- ½ cup pasta

- 1 cup of water

- 1/3 cup green peas, frozen

- 1 teaspoon salt

- ¼ teaspoon minced garlic

- 1 teaspoon tomato paste

**Directions:**

6. Mx up together water, tomato paste, minced garlic, and salt.

7. Pout liquid in the instant pot. Add green peas and pasta. Mix upgently.

8. Close the lid and set Manual mode (High pressure).

9. Cook the side dish for 10 minutes. Then use quick pressurerelease.

10.         Drain ½ part of the liquid and transfer the meal into theserving bowl.s

**Nutrition value/serving:** calories 207, fat 1.6, fiber 1.4, carbs 39.1, protein 8.7

# 12. Almond Milk Millet

**Prep:** 5 minutes **Cooking:** 10 minutes**Servings:** 3

**Ingredients:**

- ½ teaspoon salt ● 1 cup millet

- 1 cup almond milk

**Directions:**

11.  Pour almond milk in the instant pot bowl.

12.  Add millet and salt.

13.  Close and seal the lid and set Manual mode (Highpressure).

14.  Cook the side dish for 10 minutes. Allow naturalpressure release.

**Nutrition value/serving:** calories 436, fat 21.9, fiber 7.4, carbs 53, protein9.2

# 13.    Stir Fried Kale

**Prep time:** 5 minutes **Cooking time:** 5 minutes

**Servings:** 4

**Ingredients:**

- 2 cup kale, chopped

- ½ teaspoon nutritional yeast

- 1 teaspoon coconut oil

- ½ teaspoon ground black pepper

- 2 tablespoon bread crumbs

- 4 tablespoons water

**Directions:**

6. Preheat instant pot on Saute mode until hot.

7. Toss coconut oil and melt it.

8. Add chopped kale and sprinkle it with

ground black pepper andnutritional yeast.

9. Add water and saute kale for 2 minutes.

10.     Then mix up kale well and sprinkle with bread crumbs.

11.     Close the lid and cook on Manual mode (high pressure) for 1 minute. Allow quick pressure release.

12.     Shake the kale well before serving.

**Nutrition value/serving:** calories 42, fat 1.3, fiber 0.8, carbs 6.3, protein

1.7

# 14.    Zoodles

**Prep time:** 10 minutes **Cooking time:** 25 minutes

**Servings:** 4

**Ingredients:**

- 2 zucchini

- ½ teaspoon salt

- ¾ cup vegetable broth

- ¼ teaspoon ground black pepper

**Directions:**

11.    Wash and trim zucchini well.

12.    With the help of the spiralizer make the zucchinizoodles.

13.    Sprinkle them with ground black pepper and salt.

14.    Transfer zoodles in the instant pot

bowl and addvegetable broth.

15.         Close and seal the lid. Set Manual

moe (high pressure)and cook meal for 1 minute.

Use natural pressure release.

**Nutrition value/serving:** calories 23, fat 0.4, fiber

1.1, carbs 3.5, protein

2.1

# 15.  Buckwheat

**Prep time:** 10 minutes **Cooking time:** 15 minutes

**Servings:** 4

**Ingredients:**

- 2 cups buckwheat

- 2.5 cup of water

- 1 tablespoon sunflower oil

- 1 teaspoon salt

- 1 tablespoon almond butter

**Directions:**

1. Pour sunflower oil in the instant pot. Add almond butter and saute the ingredients for 3 minutes on Saute mode.

2. Then add buckwheat and stir it carefully. Saute the mixture for 3minutes.

3. Add water and stir well.

4. Close and seal the lid.

5. Set manual mode (high pressure) and cook buckwheat for 4minutes.

6. Then use quick pressure release.

7. Mix up the buckwheat carefully before serving.

**Nutrition value/serving:** calories 347, fat 8.6, fiber 8.9, carbs 61.5, protein 12.1

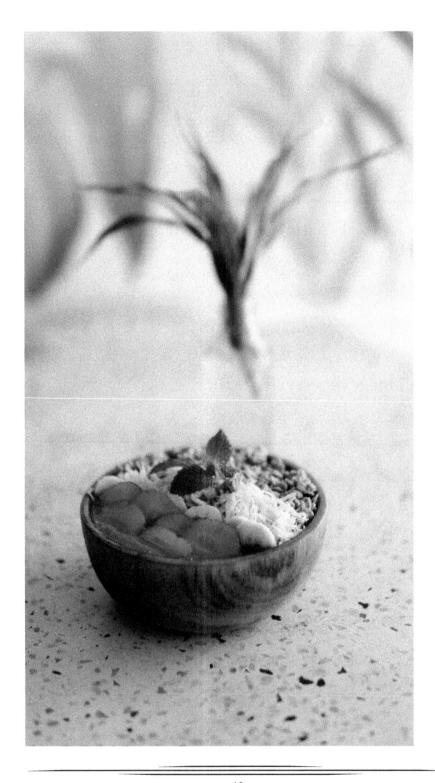

# Grains and Pasta

## 16.    Creamy Spelt Berries

**Prep time:** 5 minutes **Cooking time:** 25 minutes

**Servings:** 4

**Ingredients:**

- 1 cup spelt berries, unsoaked

- 1 teaspoon coconut oil

- 1 teaspoon salt

- 1 ½ cup vegetable broth

**Directions:**

9. Put spelt berries, coconut oil, salt, and vegetable broth in theinstant pot bowl.

10.     Close the lid and set Manual mode (high pressure).

11.     Seal the lid and cook meal for 25 minutes.

12.     Then use quick pressure release.

13.     Open the lid and stir it gently before serving.

**Nutrition value/serving:** calories 182, fat 2.4, fiber 5.5, carbs 33.1, protein

5.2

# 17.   Bulgur Salad

**Prep time:** 10 minutes **Cooking time:** 10 minutes

**Servings:** 3

**Ingredients:**

- 1/3 cup bulgur

- 1 cup of water

- 1 teaspoon salt

- 1 teaspoon tomato paste

- 1 onion, diced

- 1 bell pepper, chopped

- ½ cup tomatoes

- ½ cup arugula, chopped

- 1 teaspoon olive oil

**Directions:**

6. Pour olive oil in the instant pot. Add bell

pepper and dicedonion.

7. Mix up the vegetables and saute for 3-4 minutes.

8. After this, add bulgur, tomato paste, salt, and water. Mix it upcarefully.

9. Close the lid and cook the meal on High for 4 minutes. Then usequick pressure release.

10.     Meanwhile, in the salad bowl, mix up together choppedtomatoes and arugula.

11.     When the bulgur is cooked, open the lid and chill it tillthe room temperature.

12.     Add chilled bulgur in the salad bowl and mix up well.

**Nutrition value/serving:** calories 102, fat 2, fiber 4.7, carbs 19.9, protein3.1

# 18.    Vegan Quinoa Pilaf

**Prep time:** 10 minutes **Cooking time:** 1 minute

**Servings:** 6

**Ingredients:**

- 3 cups quinoa • 3 cups vegetable broth

- 1 teaspoon salt

- 1 teaspoon dried dill

- 1 teaspoon dried cilantro

- 1 garlic clove, peeled

- 1 teaspoon turmeric

- 1 teaspoon onion powder

- 1 tablespoon almond butter

- ¼ cup fresh parsley, chopped

**Directions:**

6. Mix up together salt, dried dill, cilantro,

turmeric, and onionpowder.

7. In the instant pot combine together dill mixture with quinoa.

8. Add garlic clove, almond butter, and vegetable broth.

9. Close and seal the lid.

10.         Set Manual mode for 1 minute (High pressure) andcook quinoa.

11.         When the time is over, use quick pressure release.

12.         Open the lid, transfer the cooked quinoa in the bowls and sprinkle with fresh parsley.

**Nutrition value/serving:** calories 353, fat 7.4, fiber 6.4, carbs 56.5, protein15.2

# 19.    Rice Garden Salad

**Prep time:** 10 minutes **Cooking time:** 6 minutes

**Servings:** 4

**Ingredients:**

- 1 cup of rice • 2 cups of water

- 1 teaspoon salt

- ½ cup spinach, chopped

- 1 cucumber, chopped

- ½ cup tomatoes, chopped

- 1 tablespoon olive oil

- 1 teaspoon chili flakes

- ½ cup green peas, canned

- 1 tablespoon fresh dill, chopped

**Directions:**

7. Cook rice: place it in the instant pot, add

salt and water. Close and seal the lid. Set manual mode (high pressure) for 6 minutes.

8. When the time is over, use quick pressure release.

9. Meanwhile, in the salad bowl mix up together chopped spinach, cucumber, tomatoes, chili flakes, olive oil, dill, and green peas.

10.      When the rice is cooked, chill it till room temperature and transfer in the salad bowl.

11.      Mix up the salad carefully and serve it warm.

**Nutrition value/serving:** calories 232, fat 4.1, fiber 2.4, carbs 43.8, protein5.3

# 20.　Lemon Pasta

**Prep:** 15 minutes **Cooking:** 15 minutes**Servings:** 4

**Ingredients:**

- 1 cup almond milk

- ½ lemon

- 12 oz spaghetti

- 3 cups of water

- 1 teaspoon wheat flour

- 1 teaspoon salt

- 1 teaspoon ground black pepper

- 1 teaspoon almond butter

- 1 tablespoon cashew, chopped

- 1 teaspoon fresh basil

**Directions:**

10.　　Cook spaghetti: place it in the

instant pot bowl, add water and salt.

11.          Close and seal the lid and cook on Manual (high pressure) for 4 minutes. Then use quick pressure release.

12.          Drain the water and transfer spaghetti in the big bowl.

13.          After this, pour almond milk in the instant pot bowl.

14.          Add wheat flour, ground black pepper, and juice from ½ lemon.

15.          Stir it gently and cook on Saute mode for 10 minutes. Stir it constantly.

16.          When the liquid starts to be thick, add cooked spaghetti and mix up well.

17.          Switch off the instant pot and

close the lid.

18.      Let the pasta rest for 2-3 minutes or until it is servingtime. Garnish spaghetti with chopped cashew.

**Nutrition value/serving:** calories 426, fat 19.6, fiber 2.1, carbs 52.9,

protein 12.4

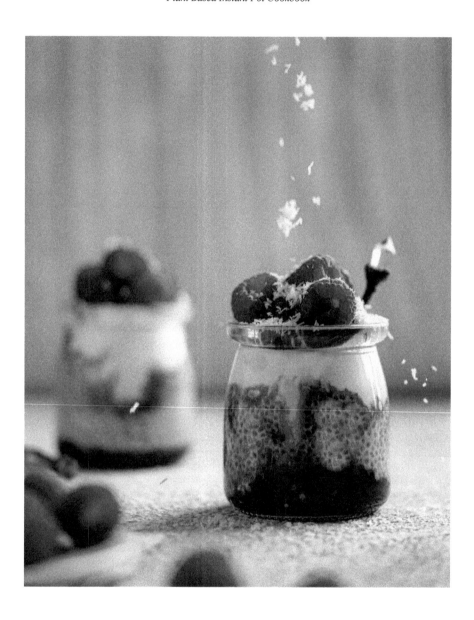

# Beans and Lentils

## 21.    Lentil Ragout

**Prep time:** 15 minutes **Cooking time:** 15 minutes

**Servings:** 4

**Ingredients:**

- 1 tomato, roughly chopped

- 2 oz celery, chopped

- 1 carrot, chopped

- 1 cup lentils

- 1 ½ cup vegetable broth

- 1 teaspoon salt

- 1 teaspoon oregano

- 1 teaspoon chili flakes

- 2 teaspoons olive oil

- 1 teaspoon tomato paste

**Directions:**

1. Pour olive oil in the instant pot and set Saute mode.

2. Add chopped celery, carrot, and mix up the ingredients. Sautethem for 5 minutes,

3. Then add tomato and lentils. Stir and cook for 3 minutes more.

4. After this, sprinkle the mixture with salt, oregano, and chiliflakes.

5. Add tomato paste and vegetable broth. Stir it until homogenous.

6. Close and seal the lid. Set Manual or High-pressure mode and cook ragout for 5 minutes.

7. Then allow natural pressure release for 10 minutes.

8. Open the lid and transfer cooked ragout into the bowls. Do notstir it anymore.

**Nutrition value/serving:** calories 209, fat 2.9, fiber 16, carbs 33, protein

12.9

# 22.    Lentil Mash

**Prep time:** 10 minutes **Cooking time:** 8 minutes

**Servings:** 4

**Ingredients:**

- 2 cup lentils

- 3 cups of water

- ½ cup tomato sauce

- ½ cup kale, chopped

**Directions:**

1. Place all the ingredients in the instant pot. Close and seal the lid.

2. Set High-pressure mode and cook the mass for 8 minutes.

3. After this, use quick pressure release and open the lid.

4. Use the hand blender to blend the mixture until you get mash.

5. Transfer the mash into the serving bowls. It is recommended to eat the meal until it is warm.

**Nutrition value/serving:** calories 350, fat 1.1, fiber 29.9, carbs 60.2,

protein 25.4

# 23.    Red Lentil Dal

**Prep:** 15 minutes **Cooking:** 10 minutes**Servings:** 3

## Ingredients:

- 1 cup red lentils 2 cups of water

- 1 tablespoon coconut oil ½ teaspoon cumin

- 1 tablespoon garlic, diced

- ½ chipotle pepper, chopped

- 1 tomato, chopped

- 1 teaspoon ground coriander

- ¾ teaspoon ground nutmeg

- 1 teaspoon salt

- ½ teaspoon chili powder

## Directions:

1. Preheat instant pot on Saute mode and add coconut oil. Melt it.

2. Add tomato, chipotle pepper, and diced garlic. Stir it and sautefor 3 minutes.

3. After this, add cumin, ground coriander, nutmeg, salt, and chili powder. Mit it up and cook for 2 minutes more.

4. Then add red lentils and water.

5. Close and seal the lid. Cook lentil dal for 5 minutes on Manualmode.

6. Then allow natural pressure release for 10 minutes.

7. Open the lid and stir the meal. Season it with salt or any otherspices if needed.

**Nutrition value/serving:** calories 281, fat 5.6, fiber 20.2, carbs 41.6,protein 17.2

## 24.    Lentil Tomato Salad

**Prep time:** 10 minutes **Cooking time:** 7 minutes

**Servings:** 5

**Ingredients:**

- 2 cups baby spinach

- 1 cup lentils

- 2 cups of water

- 1 teaspoon salt

- 1 teaspoon ground black pepper

- 3 tomatoes, chopped

- 1 red onion, sliced

- 2 tablespoons olive oil

- 1 tablespoon lemon juice

**Directions:**

1. Cook lentils: mix up lentils, water, and

salt. Transfer the mixturein the instant pot.

2. Close and seal the lid and cook on Manual for 7 minutes. Thenuse quick pressure release.

3. Meanwhile, make all the remaining preparations: combine together baby spinach with tomatoes, and red onion in the salad bowl.

4. Sprinkle with lemon juice, olive oil, and ground black pepper.Don't stir the salad.

5. Chill the cooked lentils till the room temperature and add in thesalad bowl.

6. Mix up the cooked meal carefully and serve it warm.

**Nutrition value/serving:** calories 210, fat 6.3, fiber 13.5, carbs 28.8,protein 11.2

# 25.    **Cabbage Rolls with Lentils**

**Prep time:** 15 minutes **Cooking time:** 21 minutes

**Servings:** 4

**Ingredients:**

- 9 oz cabbage, petals

- ½ cup lentils

- 1 onion, diced

- 1 carrot, diced

- 1 cup of water

- 1 teaspoon salt

- 1 teaspoon ground black pepper

- ½ cup tomato juice ¼ cup almond milk

- ½ teaspoon cayenne pepper

**Directions:**

1. Put lentils and water in the instant pot.

2. Add diced onion and carrot. Close and seal the lid. Cook the ingredients for 6 minutes on High-pressure mode.

3. Then open the lid and transfer lentil mixture in the bowl.

4. Add salt, ground black pepper, and mix it up.

5. Fill the cabbage petals with the mixture and roll them.

6. Place the cabbage rolls in the instant pot. Add tomato juice andalmond milk.

7. Sprinkle the meal with cayenne pepper and close the lid.

8. Cook it on Saute mode for 15 minutes.

9. Chill the meal for 10-15 minutes before

serving.

**Nutrition value/serving:** calories 160, fat 4, fiber

10.5, carbs 24.8, protein

8.1

# Soup and Stews

## 26.    Summer Stew

**Prep:** 15 minutes **Cooking:** 7 minutes**Servings:** 6

**Ingredients:**

- 1 eggplant, chopped roughly

- 1 cup bok choy, chopped

- 1 cup spinach, chopped

- ½ cup fresh cilantro, chopped

- 1 red onion, cut into petals

- 2 sweet peppers, chopped

- ½ cup of rice

- 5 cups vegetable broth

- 1 teaspoon salt

- 1 teaspoon thyme

- 1 teaspoon dried parsley

**Directions:**

9. Put eggplant, bok choy, spinach, cilantro, onion, and sweetpeppers in the instant pot.

10.     Add rice, vegetable broth, salt, thyme, and driedparsley.

11.     Mix up the vegetables with the help of the spoon. Closeand seal the lid.

12.     Set Manual mode (high pressure) and cook the stew for7 minutes.

13.     When the time is over, allow natural pressure release for10 minutes.

14.     Mix up the stew before serving.

**Nutrition value/serving:** calories 131, fat 1.6, fiber 4.2, carbs 22.9, protein6.9

# 27. Texas Stew

**Prep time:** 10 minutes **Cooking time:** 5 minutes

**Servings:** 2

**Ingredients:**

- ¼ cup green chili, canned, chopped
- ½ cup tomatoes, canned, diced
- ½ teaspoon salt
- 1/3 cup corn kernels, frozen
- ½ cup potatoes, chopped
- ½ cup kidney beans, canned
- ½ cup almond milk
- 1 teaspoon dried parsley

**Directions:**

12. Combine together all the ingredients in the instant pot.

13.         Close and seal the lid.

14.         Cook stew on Manual mode for 5 minutes. After this,allow natural pressure release for 5 minutes.

15.         Chill the stew till the room temperature.

16.         Transfer the stew in the serving bowls.

**Nutrition value/serving:** calories 359, fat 15.2, fiber 10.5, carbs 46, protein 13.6

# 28.    Soybean Stew

**Prep time:** 20 minutes **Cooking time:** 20 minutes

**Servings:** 4

**Ingredients:**

- 1 cup soybeans, soaked

- ¼ cup tomatoes, chopped

- 3 cups of water

- 1 teaspoon mustard

- 1 zucchini, chopped

- 1 tablespoon soy sauce

- 1 jalapeno pepper, sliced

- 3 oz vegan Parmesan, grated

**Directions:**

9. Place soybeans and tomatoes in the instant

pot.

10.      Add mustard, zucchini, soy sauce, jalapeno pepper, andclose the lid.

11.      Set Manual mode (High pressure) and cook the stew for20 minutes.

12.      Then allow natural pressure release for 20 minutes.

13.      Transfer the cooked stew in the serving bowls and topwith grated cheese.

**Nutrition value/serving:** calories 289, fat 9.6, fiber 5.3, carbs 21.2, protein 26.8

# 29.   Iranian Stew

**Prep:** 15 minutes **Cooking:** 6 minutes**Servings:** 4

**Ingredients:**

- 1 cup parsley, chopped

- ½ cup fresh cilantro, chopped

- ½ cup spinach, chopped

- ½ cup kale, chopped • ½ lime

- 1 eggplant, chopped

- 1 yellow onion, chopped

- 1 cup red kidney beans, canned

- 2 cups vegetable broth

- 1 teaspoon harissa • 2 teaspoons paprika

- 1 tablespoon almond butter

**Directions:**

    7. Put parsley, cilantro, spinach, kale, and

chopped onion in theinstant pot.

8. Add red kidney beans, vegetable broth, paprika, harissa, andalmond butter.

9. Add eggplant.

10. Close and seal the lid.

11. Cook the stew for 6 minutes in Manual mode. Afterthis, allow natural pressure release for 10 minutes.

12. Open the lid and mix up the stew carefully.

13. It is recommended to serve stew warm.

**Nutrition value/serving:** calories 259, fat 4.2, fiber 13.4, carbs 42.7,protein 16.2

# 30.    Ratsherrenpfanne

**Prep time:** 10 minutes **Cooking time:** 10 minutes

**Servings:** 2

**Ingredients:**

- 1 cup broccoli florets

- 1 cup portobello mushrooms, chopped

- ½ cup coconut cream

- ½ cup of water

- 1 teaspoon ground black pepper

- 1 teaspoon chili pepper

- 1 teaspoon corn starch

- ½ onion, diced

- 1 teaspoon olive oil

**Directions:**

8. Preheat olive oil on saute mode.

9. Add diced onion and cook it for 3-5 minutes or until lightbrown.

10. Add broccoli florets, chopped mushrooms, water, ground black pepper, chili pepper, and corn starch. Mix up the mixturewell.

11. Close and seal the lid.

12. Set Manual mode and cook the stew for 7 minutes. Usequick pressure release.

13. Open the lid and mix up the stew well with the help ofthe spatula.

14. Chill the stew till the room temperature before serving.

**Nutrition value/serving:** calories 202, fat 17, fiber 3.8, carbs 12.5, protein

4.2

# Main Dishes

## 31.   Stuffed Mini Pumpkins

**Prep time:** 30 minutes **Cooking time:** 60 minutes

**Servings:** 4

**Ingredients:**

- 2 mini pumpkin squash, trimmed, cleaned from flesh and seeds

- ½ cup chickpeas, canned

- 1 teaspoon tomato paste

- 1 cup of rice, cooked

- ½ cup fresh parsley, chopped

- 2 tablespoons almond yogurt

- 1 teaspoon chili flakes

- 1 teaspoon salt

- 1 teaspoon peanuts, chopped

- 1 teaspoon olive oil

**Directions:**

14.     In the mixing bowl combine together tomato paste and almond yogurt. Whisk the mixture.

15.     Add chili flakes, salt, peanuts, rice, parsley, and chickpeas. Mix up the mixture well.

16.     Fill the pumpkins with rice mixture. Add olive oil and wrap them into the foil.

17.     Place the mini pumpkins in the instant pot.

18.     Close and seal the lid.

19.        Set Manual mode (high pressure) and cook a meal for60 minutes.

20.        Then allow natural pressure release for 20 minutesmore.

21.        Open the lid, discard foil from the pumpkins and transfer meal on the serving plates.

**Nutrition value/serving:** calories 511, fat 4.1, fiber 6.3, carbs 41.7, protein 10.8

## 32.    Nut Loaf

**Prep time:** 15 minutes **Cooking time:** 20 minutes

**Servings:** 8

**Ingredients:**

- 1 teaspoon coconut oil

- 1 teaspoon avocado oil

- 3 oz yellow onion, diced

- 3 oz celery stalk, chopped

- 1 teaspoon garlic, diced

- 1 cup mushrooms, chopped

- ½ jalapeno pepper, chopped

- 3 oz carrot, grated

- 1 cup walnuts, chopped

- ½ cup lentils, cooked

- 1 teaspoon salt

- 1 teaspoon flax meal

- 2 tablespoons water

- ½ cup wheat flour

- 1 tablespoon Italian seasoning

- 1 cup water, for cooking

**Directions:**

13.  Preheat instant po t on saute mode.

14.  When it is hot, add avocado oil, diced onion, andmushrooms.

15.  Cook the vegetables for 5 minutes, stir them from timeto time.

16.  Then add a chopped celery stalk and mix up. Cook the mixture for 5 minutes more.

17.     Transfer the cooked vegetables into the mixing bowl.

18.     Add coconut oil, jalapeno pepper, grated carrot, walnuts, lentils, salt, and flour. Mix it up.

19.     In the separated bowl, mix up together flax meal and 2 tablespoons of water. The egg substitutor is cooked.

20.     Add the flax meal mixture into the lentils mixture.

21.     Then add Italian seasoning and mix up carefully. In the end, you should get soft but a homogenous mixture. Add more wheat flour if needed.

22.     Place the loaf mixture in the

boiling bag and seal it.

23.      Pour water in the instant pot. Add

sealed loaf.

24.      Close and seal the instant pot lid.

25.      Set Manual mode (high pressure)

and cook loaf for 6 minutes. Then allow natural

pressure release for 10 minutes more.

26.      Remove the boiling bag from the

instant pot and take loaf.

27.      Chill the loaf for 1-2 hours and

only after this, slice it.

**Nutrition value/serving:** calories 193, fat 9.8, fiber

5.8, carbs 17.8, protein

8.3

# 33.    **Fragrant Spring Onions**

**Prep time:** 15 minutes **Cooking time:** 5 minutes

**Servings:** 4

**Ingredients:**

- 1-pound spring onions

- 1 tablespoon avocado oil

- ½ teaspoon ground cumin

- 1 teaspoon dried cilantro

- ½ teaspoon salt

- 1 tablespoon lemon juice

**Directions:**

13.    Wash and trim the spring onions. Then cut themlengthwise.

14.    Sprinkle them with the dried cilantro, cumin, salt, andlemon juice.

15.     Shake well and leave for 10 minutes to marinate.

16.     Meanwhile, preheat instant pot on saute mode until hot.

17.     Add avocado oil.

18.     After this, add spring onions and cook them on Saute mode for 2 minutes from each side.

19.     Then sprinkle the vegetables with remaining lemon juice marinade and cook for 1 minute more. The spring onions are cooked when the tender but not soft.

**Nutrition value/serving:** calories 43, fat 0.8, fiber 3.2, carbs 8.7, protein

2.2

## 34.    Beet Steaks

**Prep time:** 10 minutes **Cooking time:** 27 minutes

**Servings:** 2

**Ingredients:**

- 2 red beets, peeled

- 1 portobello mushroom, chopped

- 1 white onion, sliced

- 1 teaspoon thyme

- 1 teaspoon olive oil

- 2 tablespoons red wine

**Directions:**

12.    Slice every beet onto 4 slices.

13.    Then sprinkle every beet slice with thyme.

14.    Preheat instant pot well and pour

olive oil inside.

15.      Set Saute mode, add mushrooms and sliced onion. Saute the vegetables for 3 minutes. Stir them from time to time.

16.      Transfer the cooked vegetables into the mixing bowl.

17.      Then add sliced beets in the instant pot.

18.      Add red wine and close the lid.

19.      Saute the steaks for 15 minutes.

20.      After this, add mushrooms and onion. Mix up theingredients gently.

21.      Close the lid and cook for 10 minutes more.

22.      When the time is over, switch off

the instant pot andopen the lid.

23.        Transfer the cooked beet steaks on the plates and top with the mushroom and wine sauce.

**Nutrition value/serving:** calories 110, fat 2.6, fiber 3.9, carbs 17.3, protein

3.9

# 35.    Stuffed Figs

**Prep time:** 10 minutes **Cooking time:** 2 minutes

**Servings:** 4

**Ingredients:**

- 4 figs

- ½ teaspoon brown sugar

- 3 tablespoons water

- ¼ teaspoon ground cinnamon

- 4 teaspoons cashew butter

- 1 pinch ground cardamom

- ½ cup water, for cooking

**Directions:**

19.     Crosscut the figs and remove a small amount of figflesh.

20.     Then mix up together cashew

butter, ground cinnamon,and ground cardamom.

21.       Fill the figs with the cashew butter mixture.

22.       Then place them in the instant pot pan.

23.       Sprinkle the figs with water and sugar.

24.       Pour ½ cup of water in the instant pot and insert trivet.

25.       Place pan with figs on the trivet.

26.       Close and seal the lid.

27.       Set Manual mode (high pressure) and cook figs for 2 minutes. Then use quick pressure release.

28.       Open the lid and pour the figs

with the sweet juice fromthem.

29.      The main dish should be served

hot or warm.

**Nutrition value/serving:** calories 81, fat 2.8, fiber

2.1, carbs 14.1, protein

1.6

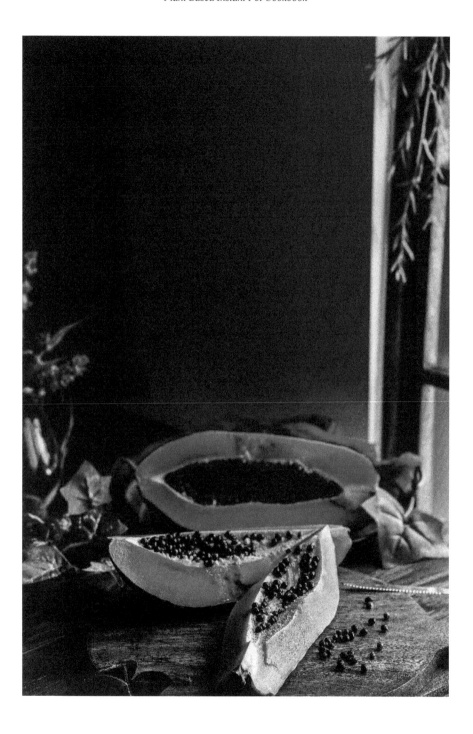

# Snacks and Appetizers

## 36.    Crunchy Artichoke Hearts

**Prep time:** 15 minutes **Cooking time:** 10 minutes

**Servings:** 2

**Ingredients:**

- 1/3 cup artichoke hearts, canned

- ½ cup panko bread crumbs

- ¼ cup almond milk

- 1 tablespoon flax meal

- 1 teaspoon paprika

- 2 tablespoons sesame oil

**Directions:**

16.    Whisk together almond milk and
       flax meal.

17.      Add paprika and stir well.

18.      Then dip artichoke hearts into the almond milk mixtureand coat in the panko bread crumbs.

19.      Pour sesame oil in the instant pot.

20.      Preheat it on saute mode.

21.      Place coated artichoke hearts in the instant pot and cookthem for 2 minutes from each side.

**Nutrition value/serving:** calories 329, fat 23.7, fiber 5.8, carbs 26.2,

protein 6

# 37. Scallion Pancakes

**Prep time:** 10 minutes **Cooking time:** 5 minutes

**Servings:** 4

**Ingredients:**

- ½ cup scallions, chopped

- 2 tablespoons flax meal

- 4 tablespoons water

- 1 teaspoon salt

- 1 potato, peeled, boiled

- 1 tablespoon olive oil

- 1 teaspoon ground black pepper

**Directions:**

23.    Mix up together flax meal and water. Whisk it.

24.    Add chopped scallions, salt, and

ground black pepper.

25.      After this, mash potato and add it in the scallionsmixture.

26.      Stir it well.

27.      Make the balls from the mixture and press them to getpancake shape.

28.      Pour olive oil in the instant pot. Preheat it on Sautemode.

29.      Add scallions pancakes and cook them for 2 minutesfrom each side.

**Nutrition value/serving:** calories 83, fat 4.8, fiber 2.4, carbs 9.7, protein

1.9

# 38. Mushroom Arancini

**Prep time:** 10 minutes **Cooking time:** 6 minutes

**Servings:** 8

**Ingredients:**

- ½ cup mushrooms, chopped, fried

- ½ cup of rice, cooked

- ½ onion, minced

- ¼ teaspoon minced garlic

- 4 oz vegan Parmesan, grated

- 3 tablespoons flax meal

- 5 tablespoons almond milk

- ¼ cup olive oil

- 1 cup bread crumbs

**Directions:**

20. Put chopped mushrooms, rice,

minced onion, garlic, and grated cheese in the blender.

21.        Blend the mixture for 30 seconds.

22.        After this, transfer it in the mixing bowl.

23.        In the separated bowl whisk together almond milk and flax meal.

24.        Add the flax meal mixture in the rice mixture and stir well.

25.        Pour olive oil in the instant pot and bring it to boil on Saute mode.

26.        Meanwhile, make balls from the rice mixture and coat them in the bread crumbs well.

27.        Place the mushroom balls in the

hot olive oil and cook for 3 minutes or until light

brown.

28.        Dry the snack with the paper

        towel.

**Nutrition value/serving:** calories 230, fat 10.3, fiber

1.9, carbs 23.9,

protein 9.4

# 39.    **Coated Heart of Palm**

**Prep time:** 10 minutes **Cooking time:** 25 minutes

**Servings:** 4

**Ingredients:**

- 1 cup heart of palm

- ¼ cup wheat flour

- ½ teaspoon salt

- 1 teaspoon maple syrup

- ½ teaspoon paprika

- ½ teaspoon soy sauce

- ¼ cup coconut flakes

- 2 tablespoon sesame oil

**Directions:**

23.        Mix up together wheat flour, salt, paprika, and coconutflakes.

24.      In the separated bowl, mix up together the heart ofpalm, maple syrup, and soy sauce. Stir gently.

25.      Toss the heart of palm in the coconut flakes mixture andcoat well.

26.      Pour sesame oil in the instant pot and preheat it onSaute mode.

27.      Cook coated heart of palm in the hot oil for 2 minutes. Then dry with the help of the paper towel.

28.      Serve the snack with your favorite vegan sauce.

**Nutrition value/serving:** calories 122, fat 8.8, fiber 1.7, carbs 9.7, protein 2

# 40.   Sweet Tofu Cubes

**Prep time:** 10 minutes **Cooking time:** 40 minutes

**Servings:** 2

**Ingredients:**

- 6 oz firm tofu, cubed

- 1 teaspoon mustard

- 1 teaspoon olive oil

- 1 teaspoon apple cider vinegar

- ½ teaspoon maple syrup

**Directions:**

22.     Place tofu in the instant pot.

23.     Sprinkle it with mustard, olive oil,

apple cider vinegar,and maple syrup.

24.     Mix up the mixture well.

25.     Close and seal the lid.

26.     Cook tofu cubes for 2 minutes on High-pressure mode.

27.     Then use quick pressure release.

28.     Transfer the tofu cubes on the serving plate and sprinkle with the remaining gravy.

29.     Insert a toothpick in every tofu cube.

**Nutrition value/serving:** calories 92, fat 6.4, fiber 1, carbs 3.2, protein 7.4

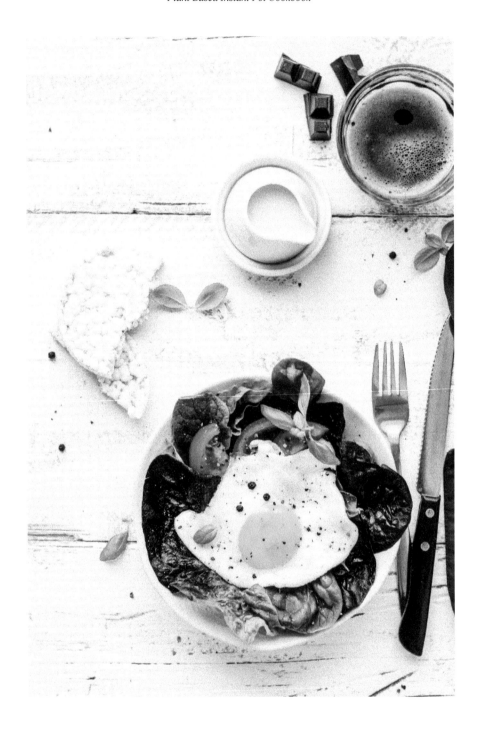

# Sauces and Fillings

## 41.   Roasted Pepper Salsa

**Prep time:** 10 minutes **Cooking time:** 5 minutes

**Servings:** 4

**Ingredients:**

- 1-pound sweet pepper, seeded

- 1 cup tomatoes, chopped

- 1 oz fresh basil

- 1 teaspoon salt

- 1 teaspoon ground black pepper

- 1 garlic clove, chopped

- 1 tablespoon balsamic vinegar

- 2 tablespoons olive oil

- 1 cup water, for cooking

# Directions:

28.       Pour water in the instant pot. Insert the trivet.

29.       Place sweet peppers on the trivet and close the lid.

30.       Cook them on Manual mode (high pressure) for 5minutes.

31.       Then use quick pressure release.

32.       Open the lid and transfer the peppers in the blender.

33.       Add tomatoes, fresh basil, salt, ground black pepper, garlic, balsamic vinegar, and olive oil.

34.       Blend the mixture for 1 minute.

35.       Transfer the cooked salsa in the

serving bowl.

**Nutrition value/serving:** calories 82, fat 7.2, fiber 1.2, carbs 4.8, protein 1

# 42.  Arugula Hummus

**Prep time:** 25 minutes **Cooking time:** 25 minutes

**Servings:** 4

**Ingredients:**

- 1 cup garbanzo beans, soaked

- 3 cups of water

- 2 cups arugula

- 1 teaspoon salt

- 1 teaspoon harissa

- 1 tablespoon olive oil

- 1 teaspoon lemon juice

- ½ teaspoon tahini

**Directions:**

29.    Cook garbanzo beans: place water and beans in the instant pot.

30.        Close and seal the lid; cook the
beans for 25 minutes, then allow natural pressure
release for 20 minutes more.

31.        After this, transfer beans and 1/3
cup of bean water inthe blender.

32.        Add arugula, salt, harissa, olive
oil, lemon juice, andtahini.

33.        Blend the mixture until smooth.

34.        Transfer arugula hummus in the
           serving bowl.

**Nutrition value/serving:** calories 223, fat 7.2, fiber
8.9, carbs 31.4, protein
10.1

# 43.    Edamole

**Prep time:** 10 minutes **Cooking time:** 8 minutes

**Servings:** 4

**Ingredients:**

- 1 cup green soybeans, soaked

- 4 cups of water

- 1 garlic clove, chopped

- ½ teaspoon ground cumin

- 1 tablespoon hot sauce

**Directions:**

25.    Place water and soybeans in the instant pot.

26.    Close and seal the lid.

27.    Cook soybeans on manual mode for 30 minutes. Thenuse quick pressure release.

28.     Drain water and transfer soybeans in the blender.

29.     Add garlic clove, ground cumin, and hot sauce.

30.     Blend the mixture for 1-2 minutes.

31.     Transfer edamole in the serving bowl.

**Nutrition value/serving:** calories 210, fat 9.3, fiber 4.4, carbs 14.5, protein 17.1

# 44.  Pizza Sauce

**Prep time:** 5 minutes **Cooking time:** 6 minutes

**Servings:** 6

**Ingredients:**

- ½ cup tomato juice

- ¼ cup almond yogurt

- 1 teaspoon minced garlic

- 1 teaspoon dried dill

- 1 teaspoon Italian seasoning

- 1 teaspoon maple syrup

- 1 teaspoon chili pepper

- 1 teaspoon olive oil

**Directions:**

23.        Pour olive oil in the instant pot.

Preheat it on Sautemode.

24.     Add   chili   pepper,   Italian seasoning, dried dill, andminced garlic.

25.     Cook the mixture for 2 minutes. Stir it.

26.     Then add maple syrup, tomato juice, and almondyogurt. Mix up the mixture.

27.     Close the lid and saute sauce for 4 minutes.

28.     Then open the lid, mix up the sauce one more time andtransfer it in the bowl.

**Nutrition value/serving:** calories 24, fat 1.4, fiber 0.2, carbs 2.8, protein

0.4

# 45.    Garlic Dip

**Prep time:** 15 minutes **Cooking time:** 5 minutes

**Servings:** 2

**Ingredients:**

- ½ cup almond milk

- ¼ cup garlic, minced

- 1 teaspoon salt

- ½ teaspoon ground black pepper

- 1 teaspoon cornflour

**Directions:**

31.    Pour almond milk in the instant

pot.

32.    Preheat it on Saute mode.

33.    Add cornflour and whisk well.

34.    Then add minced garlic, salt, and

ground black pepper.

35.     Keep whisking dip for 3 minutes more.

36.     Then switch off the instant pot and close the lid.

37.     Let the dip rest for 10-15 minutes before serving.

**Nutrition value/serving:** calories 169, fat 14.5, fiber 1.9, carbs 10.2,

protein 2.6

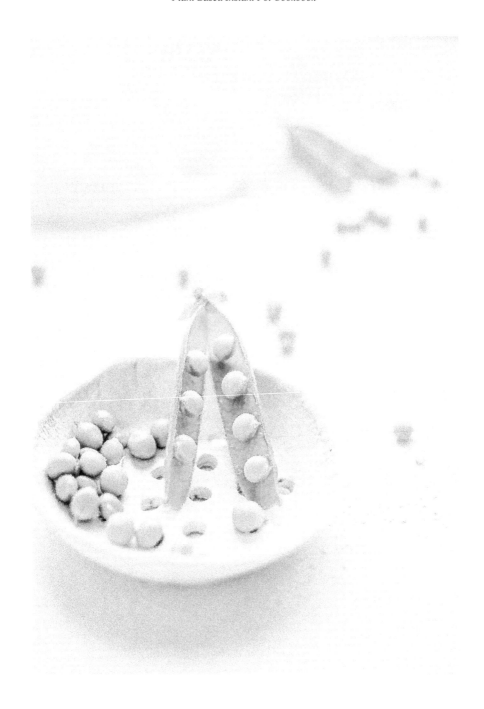

# Desserts

## 46.    Cream Pie Pudding

**Prep time:** 15 minutes **Cooking time:** 10 minutes

**Servings:** 5

**Ingredients:**

- 2 cups cashew milk

- 1 tablespoon vanilla extract

- 1 tablespoon corn flour

- 1 teaspoon cornstarch

- 4 oz vegan raw chocolate, chopped

- ½ cup of coconut milk

- 1/3 cup sugar

- 2 tablespoons coconut flakes

**Directions:**

20.        Mix up together cashew milk,

vanilla extract, corn flour,cornstarch, and sugar.

21.        Pour the liquid in the blender and blend it for 15seconds.

22.        Preheat the instant pot on Saute mode until hot.

23.        Pour cashew milk mixture in the instant pot. Boil theliquid until it thickens.

24.        Then pour the pudding in the bowl.

25.        After this, clean the instant pot and place raw chocolateinside.

26.        Add coconut milk and saute the mixture untilhomogenous.

27.        Then make the last preparations of the dessert: take the glass jars and pour small

inside of the cashew milk pudding inside.

28.     Then   add   melted   chocolate
        mixture.

29.     Repeat the steps until you use all
        the mixtures.

30.     Chill the pudding.

**Nutrition value/serving:** calories 267, fat 16.2, fiber

8.1, carbs 28.6,

protein 1.5

# 47.   Banana Cake

**Prep:** 15 minutes **Cooking:** 7 minutes**Servings:** 4

## Ingredients:

- 5 bananas, peeled ● 6 oz rice flour

- 1 teaspoon vanilla extract

- 1 tablespoon brown sugar

- 1 tablespoon peanut butter

- Cooking spray ● 1 cup water, for cooking

## Directions:

19.     Chop the bananas and place them in the mixing bowl.

20.     Mash the fruits with the help of the fork.

21.     After this, add rice flour, vanilla extract, and brownsugar.

22.      Mix up the mixture well.

23.      Spray the springform pan with cooking spray and pourbanana mixture in it.

24.      Pour water in the instant pot, insert trivet; placespringform pan on the trivet.

25.      Close and seal the lid. Cook the cake for 7 minutes.

26.      Then allow natural pressure release for 10 minutes.

27.      Spread the cooked cake with peanut butter and cut intoslices.

**Nutrition value/serving:** calories 322, fat 3.1, fiber 5.1, carbs 70.9, protein

5.1

# 48.    Carambola in Chai Syrup

**Prep time:** 15 minutes **Cooking time:** 6 minutes

**Servings:** 2

**Ingredients:**

- 2 cups carambola, sliced

- ½ cup chai syrup

- 1/3 cup water

- ¼ teaspoon ground ginger

**Directions:**

28.    In the instant pot mix up together chai syrup and water.

29.    Add ground ginger.

30.    Set Saute mode and cook the liquid for 5 minutes.

31.    Then add sliced carambola stir

gently and cook for 1 minute more.

32.        Switch off the instant pot and let

carambol soak thesyrup.

**Nutrition value/serving:** calories 52, fat 0.4, fiber

3.1, carbs 11.9, protein

1.1

# 49.    Semolina Pudding with Mango

**Prep time:** 15 minutes **Cooking time:** 10 minutes

**Servings:** 4

**Ingredients:**

- 2 cups almond milk

- ½ cup semolina

- 4 oz mango puree

- 3 tablespoons brown sugar

- 1 teaspoon vanilla extract

- 1 teaspoon coconut oil

**Directions:**

22.      Pour almond milk in the instant pot and preheat it onSaute mode.

23.      When it starts to boil, add semolina, brown sugar, andvanilla extract.

24.    Bring it to boil again. Stir well.

25.    Then close the lid and switch off the instant pot.

26.    Leave it for 10 minutes.

27.    After this, add coconut oil and stir well.

28.    Place mango puree in the serving bowls.

29.    Add semolina pudding over the puree.

**Nutrition value/serving:** calories 404, fat 30, fiber 3.7, carbs 32.1, protein 5.5

# 50.    **Walnut Sweets**

**Prep time:** 5 minutes **Cooking time:** 5 minutes

**Servings:** 4

**Ingredients:**

- 1 cup walnuts kernels

- 4 oz vegan raw chocolate, chopped

- ¾ cup almond milk

**Directions:**

21.      Preheat instant pot on Saute mode

until hot.

22.      Add chopped raw chocolate and

cook it for 2 minutes.

23.      When it is melted, add almond

milk and whisk untilhomogenous.

24.      Then coat the walnut kernels in

the chocolate mixture.

25.        Line the tray with the baking

paper.

26.        Transfer the coated chocolate

walnuts on the preparedtray. Let the sweets dry.

27.        Stor the walnut sweets in the

closed paper box.

**Nutrition value/serving:** calories 459, fat 40.3, fiber

12.2, carbs 19.8,

protein 9.6

# Conclusion

Presently, the world is divided into people who support veganism and those who are against the complete abandonment of animal products. Hope this book could dispel your stereotypes that vegetarian food is monotonous and not tasty. If you have already read some pages of the cookbook, you know that it includes hundreds of magnificent and very easy to cook recipes. It is possible to say that this vegan recipe guide can be a good gift to everyone who loves delicious food. These days veganism is a sought-after way of life. More often people refuse to consume all types of meat and dairy products and limit yourself with fruits, vegetables, and another produces. It is true that thanks to the vegan lifestyle you can improve your health and feel much better. Scientifically proved that total refusing from any type of meat and dairy products can help fight with Type

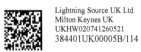

Lightning Source UK Ltd.
Milton Keynes UK
UKHW020741260521
384401UK00005B/114

9 781802 891751